Juice Fasting Made Simple

Your Guide to Juicy Tips and Tricks

Sharon E. Johnson

Please Note

The content of this book is for general informational purposes only. It is not meant to be used, nor should it be used, to diagnose or treat any medical condition or to replace the services of your physician or other healthcare provider. The advice and strategies contained in the book may not be suitable for all readers. Please consult your healthcare provider for any questions that you may have about your own medical situation. Neither the author, publisher, IIN, nor any of their employees or representatives guarantees the accuracy of information in this book or its usefulness to a particular reader, nor are they responsible for any damages or negative consequences that may result from any treatment, action taken, or inaction by any person reading or following the information in this book.

For information, contact Sharon Johnson at info@rawandawesome.com

To contact the publisher, visit
CreateSpace.com

To contact the author, visit
RawandAwesome.com

ISBN-10: 1539857557
ISBN-13: 978-1539857556

Printed in the United States of America

DEDICATION

To all of you reading this book.
Remember you are loved, and you are love.
It begins with you.
I Am That, I AM.

Be the change that you wish to see in the world - Gandhi

ACKNOWLEDGMENTS

Working on this book has been a rewarding experience. The ability to assist others through their juice fasting experience has been one of my greatest pleasures.

This book would not exist without those that inspired me, cheered me on, and supported me throughout the years. I would like to acknowledge in particular:

God for giving me the discipline and dedication to take on this book writing challenge and for giving me strength. I am thankful for your guidance through this journey to health and happiness and for the will to complete many juice fasts!

My great friend and official editor Khandra Dillard-Robinson. I appreciate your help and support on this journey and for making me sound great.

PHOTOGRAPHY

Endigo Rae, Back Cover Headshot

Kenzi Taiow, Front Cover

Introduction

It is not by chance that you desire to improve your health and wellness. Like most health-conscious enthusiasts, I know the desire to feel better and achieve our highest potential - both physically and spiritually - are the driving forces behind juice fasting and living a raw foods diet.

As it is in the natural, so it is in the spiritual. Our world in its current state is a direct reflection of where we are collectively in the spiritual realm. We begin to transform our lives through the belief that we have the power to change. Thus we transform the world around us by our own personal transformation.

Do you desire to lose weight? Eat high vibrational foods. Fast intermittently. Unwanted pounds will be eliminated. Do you desire to be more spiritually balanced? Complete a juice fast. Not only will you be more spiritually aware, but you will also be led to where your spirit desires to be. Maybe you just want to be healthier in general? Ingesting vibrant, nutrient-dense foods and juices will give your body the nutrition it needs to heal and repair itself.

The purpose of this book is to:

• Encourage you in this journey to a healthier lifestyle

• Provide a safe non-judgmental environment

• Inform and point you to valuable resources such as books, websites, blogs, life centers, etc.

• Provide assistance with mental, emotional, and physical obstacles

• Remind you that your participation is essential. You create your day, and you choose how to respond situations

• Let you know that you are not alone. Sometimes we feel like our story is singularly unique when, in reality, we are a collective body going through similar experiences. It is up to us to encourage each other, lovingly, in a safe space with no judgment

What is Juice Fasting?

Juice fasting is the act of limiting your diet to freshly extracted juice from fruit, green leafy vegetables, herbs, and other produce.

Fasting is known for limiting the amounts of juice and/or food one ingests. For the purposes of this book, the definition of juice fasting is simple: eliminating all foods and beverages unless in liquid form or able to be completely dissolved. (This includes eliminating pulp.)

Fad or not, juicing has become increasingly popular. Critics are of the opinion that juicing is just the current craze, is extreme, cannot be maintained, and hinders fasters from nutrients and needed fiber. However, juicing has been around for centuries and even discussed in the *Essene Gospel of Peace Book 1* of the Dead Sea scrolls.

Juice fasting can occur in several variations. Some fasts exchange one or two daily meals for juice. Another variation is to fast on juice until dinner or dusk. Some people choose to safely eliminate solids from their diet for a length of time whether it be an entire day or 120 days. The amount of liquid ingested varies from limited ounces to more than a gallon which supports light activity throughout the day.

The reasons people juice fast are also varied. Individuals may decide to fast for spiritual purposes, detoxification, weight loss, or other reasons.

Drinking freshly extracted juice is highly recommended as its nutritional value is at its peak, and its enzymes are still active. Enzymes, present in living and raw juices and foods, aid in the absorption of vital nutrients. Loss of these enzymes, and the oxidation of produce can compromise the flavor, color, and nutritional value of juice. Enzymes are necessary as the body only has a limited amount of digestive enzymes. As the body digests food and beverages, it pulls from its réservoir of enzymes. For optimal nutritional value, it is recommended to ingest fresh juice immediately.

Food generally loses nutritional value due to pasteurization and oxidation which can impact up to 80% of its nutritional value. Although freshly extracted juice is recommended, it is possible to fast successfully on the bottled juice that is not from concentrate. Fasting with juice from concentrate should be used as a last resort.

Reasons to Do a Juice Fast

Juicing is able to alleviate and reverse common ailments such as high blood pressure, diabetes, eczema, and obesity. Juicing helps the body to reboot itself, remove toxicity, regain energy, and have glowing skin. It makes you want to connect with nature and can increase your overall health, happiness, and longevity.

Some of the benefits of juice fasting are:

1. Juicing boosts your immune system and helps it battle the flu, colds, and seasonal allergies

2. It is one of the fastest ways to rid your body of toxins

3. You receive the health benefits of live enzymes and the highest possible nutritional value from the juice

4. It is an easy way to get your recommended servings of fruits and vegetables

5. Fresh juice is not pasteurized like most store bought juices

6. You have control over the ingredients - whether they are conventional, organic, local, seasonal, etc.

7. Juicing can offer relief from common ailments and diseases like headaches and high blood pressure

8. Replacing a meal with fresh juice can help you lose weight without depriving your body of the nutrients it needs

9. Juicing can boost your energy level without the crash that caffeine and sugar sometimes cause

10. Juice fasting is able to reach your body on the cellular level, allowing your digestive system to take a break, and turn your body's attention to healing

11. The ability to get the maximum nutrients the earth provided without eating pounds of fruit and vegetables

12. Improved digestion and the enzymes needed to digest food

13. Finding the fountain of youth and improved skin appearance

14. Heightened spiritual awareness

What About Smoothies?

You can do modified fasts with success. Determine what your goal is and then decide what is right for you.

Juicing detoxes you on a cellular level. It allows your body to rest from digestion and focus on healing. You feel lighter. You feel the healing and detox effects faster. Nutrients are absorbed by the body faster.

Smoothies also allow your body to detox. The detox process and results are slower but can still be powerful if you use many healing vegetables and a little fruit. Smoothies are denser feeling per ounce and keep you full longer. They can be faster and easier to prepare with less prep and cleaning time. Because of the amount of fiber they contain, they allow for more elimination. You also have less pre- and post-detox transition time.

Toxicity and Detoxing

Fasting gives your body the opportunity to release toxins. Toxins come from pollution in the air, pesticides, water, household products, personal care products, food, stress, and even harmful thoughts.

Fasting gives the body the opportunity to reset itself. Joshua Rosenthal of the Institute for Integrative Nutrition frequently says that, given half a chance, our body will heal itself. Digesting solid foods slows down the body's opportunity to work on other organs. When your digestion system is at rest, your body has the chance to take the ingested nutrients and work on tissue, organs, and cells.

Many detoxes work. However, juicing works because the liquid is more readily absorbed than foods ingested on other programs. Juice is able to be digested at a cellular level. The juice that is ingested is nutrient dense and has the building blocks your body needs to heal itself.

My Story

I grew up in sunny Arizona eating a Standard American Diet - protein, starch, veggie, dairy, and fruit. Although my mom insisted on following the "Food Pyramid," I somehow found a way to duck out of fresh fruit and vegetables (with lemons, grapefruit, and pickles being the exceptions).

I remember hearing my mom say, "You have to put something green on your plate." My diet consisted of breakfast with cereal (I loved Cream of Wheat with milk), toast, bacon or sausage, and orange juice. Lunch from the school cafeteria was typically sandwiches, a few vegetables, and always plenty of milk to drink.

My weekend lunches were Mexican food. "Heavy on the sour cream and cheese, please!" I enjoyed my favorite snacks: nachos, grilled cheese sandwiches, cheese crisps, cookies, and milk. Dinner generally was a protein, green vegetable, and starches - one with some type of cheese sauce. Imagine my plate filled with fish and fries, spaghetti, smothered chicken, meatloaf, potatoes, rice, and bread.

I battled with my weight throughout my school years. Along with poor food choices, it not only affected my health but my happiness, self-esteem, feelings of self-worth, and connection with myself.

By high school, I began to develop a delayed allergen reaction to dairy. I could no longer eat any raw fruits or vegetables other than lettuce.

When I got to college, I became aware of the possible consequences of my health and diet. My family has a history of diabetes, hypertension, and breast cancer. I knew if I continued down the same path of diet and lifestyle, I would be on medication by the time I reached my mid-30s or soon after.

My life and livelihood were dependent on finding a diet plan and lifestyle that worked for me. I spent over a decade sampling various menus and plans. I tried high protein diets, elimination diets, the Cabbage Soup Diet, the Grapefruit Diet, a vegetable soup diet, and other trends. I lost weight on each plan. However, during and after the diet, I was always left feeling deprived, irritable, tired, and I gained back more weight than I lost. It was a vicious and often depressing cycle.

The diets I attempted did not teach me how to eat to live and rarely encouraged exercise. The search continued. Finally, the building blocks of a healthy vibrant life came to me. Out of frustration, and a discussion of health with a girlfriend, I learned about the Raw Foods Diet.

My friend mentioned she was interested in fasting for life by eating raw fruits and vegetables. I began to do research. I learned about the Raw Food Diet also known as the Sunfood Diet, Raw Foodism, or Raw Vegan Diet. I was utterly intrigued by what I read in books and online. People were not only losing weight, but they were also battling illness and reversing diseases such as cancer, heart disease, diabetes, Multiple Sclerosis, and seeing positive impacts in their moods and happiness. There were other significant effects as well: mental clarity, improved skin, aches disappearing, reduction in allergies and candida, and more.

I was learning about the possibilities of health and wellness by following this one diet and lifestyle. This Raw Foods Diet resonated with me.

After trying the meals several times and eliminating certain foods from my diet, not only did I regain the ability to eat fresh fruit and vegetables, but I also lost weight, had clearer skin, and increased energy. I wanted to connect with nature, and I had a new found zest for life.

I began researching the Raw Foods Diet and incorporating fresh produce into my diet on a regular basis. However, I still struggled with going back and forth from a majority raw foods diet to the Standard American Diet with emphasis on meat, dairy, and cheese. My weight bounced around like a yo-yo. I set a goal to move towards a vegan lifestyle. However, my cravings and addictions to certain foods were more than I could overcome at the time. This started me on my journey to go deeper into a raw and awesome diet and lifestyle.

As I learned about raw foods, I began to find out more about detoxification through juice fasting. I decided to incorporate juice fasting into my regimen to help reboot my body, release cravings, and prepare my body for the elimination of foods from my diet. Juicing has become a method that resonates with me on many levels - physically, emotionally, mentally, and spiritually.

My most extended juice fast was 60 days! That extended fast was one of my most rewarding accomplishments in life. I decided to do it because I was ready to reset my body on a more profound holistic level. I knew that I would reset cravings and increase my energy. I was looking forward to enhancing my mental clarity and spiritual connection.

It took a lot of discipline, research, and support from all my friends to be successful. It was the first attempt of many. I tried several times and did not make it past ten or fourteen days. There were several reasons why juice fasting was difficult for me to complete. I did not have a sense of community, I was not aware of the proper procedures to follow, and I lacked direction.

Juice fasting can be a very lonely or enriching experience. I needed something or someone to help me. At the time I completed the 60-day fast, I had just begun school at the Institute for Integrative Nutrition to become a certified holistic health coach. I had a tremendous sense of community, I had cheerleaders by my side, and I was surrounded by a wealth of health and knowledge from the school. It could not get any better.

During my juice fasting journey, I have learned a lot about what helps to ease the process financially and mentally. I was able to successfully complete my 60-day fast with several tips that I want to share with you.

My 60-Day Juice Fast

Before I completed my juice fast, I had low energy, a weakened immune system, excess weight, little mental clarity, short-term memory, and uncontrollable cravings. I wanted to use the fast as an opportunity to give up foods that were not nourishing me. As I was learning about the Raw Foods Diet, I was eating a lot of fruit and vegetables but still ingesting a lot of dairy and protein. It was challenging to give up addicting foods. I trusted that the juice fast would help me to eliminate or minimize those cravings for good.

After I completed my juice fast, not only did I lose 20 pounds, but I was told that I appeared to be reversing in age! Finding the fountain of youth made me almost more excited than the weight loss. I no longer had eczema, my skin glowed, and that youthful look in my face returned.

Around day 14 of the fast, I was able to see clearer. Everything looked brighter. I felt very light - as if I was walking 2 inches off the ground. I felt a strong urge to connect with people, animals, and nature. I not only felt better physically but I also had mental clarity and felt emotionally balanced. I was spiritually connected and learned a tremendous amount about my inner self. I was excited and happy on a regular basis.

My body began to feel like it was running optimally. I did not realize how bright and keen our senses can become. My sense of smell was heightened, and my sense of taste was enhanced. I remember, after completing the juice fast, getting a vegetable burrito that had cooked beans, fresh onions, fresh cilantro, and a tortilla wrap. The only things I could taste from the burrito were the onions and cilantro! Fruits and vegetables tasted brilliant. Everything else seemed bland, over-processed, and in need of seasoning. I almost felt like I had superpowers.

I also took the opportunity to do self-development and work on my spiritual growth. I implemented a meditation and prayer regimen. I went walking regularly. I took moments to journal reasons why I was grateful. The detox was not only about my body, but it was also about connecting with my soul.

Having a great support system, the tools, and the resources, being mentally prepared for the fast, and seeing beautiful results made my extended fast a pleasant, beautiful, and successful experience.

What You Will Get From This Book

In this book, you will receive tips on completing a fast on any budget with your busy schedule in mind. You will understand how to successfully transition into the fast, continue on the fast, and transition out safely.

You will know what to expect during the program: detox symptoms, whether or not you will be hungry, what is the right fruit to vegetable ratio, the benefits of supplements, and more.

You will have the confidence to know that you can complete a juice fast, know that each attempt is a success, and know if a fast is for you. The necessary information on how to complete the detox, with or without taking a lot of time and effort, is in the following chapters. You can complete a juicing plan whether you have a busy schedule or are traveling. You will learn what kind of fast is right for you: switching out one meal a day with a glass of juice or completing a 10-day or longer juice fast.

To make your juice fasting journey more comfortable, there is a sample 3-day plan in this book to help you get started on your juice fasting journey.

In this book, you will see the use of the word "raw" interchangeably with "living."

You will find a variety of tips and juice recipes to help you obtain your juice fasting goals.

Please take a few moments to review each chapter. It's time to get started on this raw and awesome journey!

Appliances

When preparing for juicing, the correct equipment can make for a more straightforward process. Selecting proper kitchen tools can determine the cost, time, and efficiency of your juice fast.

Most of the following recommendations are optional. Choose what works best for you and your budget. When I first started juicing, I purchased an affordable juicer that was less than $100. The brand I purchased was not very practical for extracting juice from green leafy vegetables. However, for occasional juicing, it worked. When I decided to complete an extended juice fast, I upgraded to a high-speed blender and a sprouting bag. Review your budget and how much time you have to select tools and methods that will work for you.

Juicer

This is a kitchen appliance that very few people had just a few years ago. Juicers are becoming much more common in home kitchens as people are beginning to understand and appreciate the health benefits of juicing. There are many different styles, prices, and levels of quality in the world of juicers.

There are several different ways to juice your fruits and vegetables. One way, used by masticating juicers, is primarily a slow, steady grind. This protects the vital nutrients from prolonged air exposure that can break down and reduce the juice's health benefits. Most high-end home juicers are of the masticating variety.

The other common type is the centrifugal juicer. This technology extracts juice by cutting and spinning produce at high rpms. This technique is usually not the most efficient and allows much more oxidation which impacts the longevity of the juice, resulting in slightly less nutrition.

At the higher end of the financial spectrum is the cold pressed technique. The fruits and vegetables are slowly pressed under terrific force leading to almost complete extraction of the juice. Because nothing is essentially being cut, this process has the least amount of air exposure. One negative is that the machines used to do this are generally large and highly expensive.

Citrus Juicer

Due to the fine pulp, a citrus juicer is recommended for fruit like grapefruit, oranges, lemons, and limes. You can choose from electric citrus juicers, citrus pressers, and citrus reamers. Electric juicers allow you to extract juice quickly and are convenient for juicing several citrus items in less time. However, they take more time to clean. Citrus presses are suitable for extracting juice from a few pieces of fruit and citrus reamers are reasonably priced manual juicers.

Cutting Board

A set of cutting boards is essential for juicing because they protect your counters. I recommend a cutting board made out of wood (like bamboo) or crafted from a durable, nonporous material.

Produce Drying Mat

Produce drying mats are not essential but definitely come in handy. They are incredibly absorbent and helpful while pre-washing your fruit. When using, make sure your produce is completely dry before storing. A simple, clean towel will do the trick as well (although generally not as absorbent).

Knife

A good set of knives can help you get in and out of the kitchen in no time. Different knives help to prep your variety of produce safely.

Mason Jars

Mason jars are a juicer's favorite. Choose glass jars with either metal or plastic lids. If you are not drinking your juice immediately, fill the jar to the top and seal with a little lemon juice to keep air (oxidation) out and your juice will keep longer.

Storage Containers

If you are pre-washing your produce, you will want a good set of containers. This will help your produce last longer.

Strainer/Nut Milk Bag

This is another optional item dependent on you, the juicer. If you are using a blender to juice or have a juicer that extracts pulp along with the juice, you will want to use some type of strainer.

Liquid Measuring Cups

If you like to follow recipes precisely, you may want to invest in a set of liquid measuring cups. This will help you to perfect recipes as well as help with pouring.

Measuring Spoons

Measuring spoons are an excellent tool for measuring out your daily supplements. Any set will do.

Salad Spinner

If you are pre-rinsing your leafy greens, you will want to make sure the greens are as dry as possible. A salad spinner will help to facilitate the air-drying process.

Colander

A colander is perfect for rinsing off your produce without sending it down the drain.

Vegetable Brush

A vegetable brush is used to help remove debris and wax off of your produce. Get a brush that is flexible and easy to grip.

High-Speed Blender for Juicing

When I first started juicing, I did not want to purchase an expensive juicer. My regular juicer was sufficient for extracting juice from fruit but not from green leafy vegetables. I decided to invest in a high-speed blender.

To use a high-speed blender for juicing, you need a sprouting bag also known as a nut milk bag. After blending your produce, with a little water to get started, you strain the juice through the sprouting bag into a big bowl. This method worked wonders and provided a mini arm workout as well. If you choose this option for an extended fast, you will want to soak the bag in peroxide for cleaning after each use. Consider investing in a couple of extra bags as the wringing will cause wear and tear over time.

This method proved to be useful as I was able to save hundreds of dollars on a new juicer, especially before knowing if I was going to complete an extended juice fast successfully. The pros to the process are that you can throw all of your produce in the pitcher at once, quickly do a taste test, and see if you want to add any other ingredients.

The cons of this method are multiple. Its more time consuming to extract the juice. Also, it can be messy as you are hand-wringing the juice from the sprout bag which can change the color and smell of your hands temporarily - especially if you are using carrots, beets, and garlic. In addition, the oxidation may occur faster since you are blending at high speed.

Produce for Juicing

Creating great juices is an art form. People have many questions on combining produce to make vibrant, nutritious, and delicious juice. Once you have the basics down, creating beautiful juices will be a breeze.

Keep it simple. Remember less is more. Five ingredients or less is plenty. Choose a base by picking produce that yields a high amount of liquid. Add one or two other fruits or vegetables. Lastly, as you become accustomed to the juice, add a few "super" ingredients that are more potent as well as additional cleansing properties and nutrients to your creation.

Start where you are and enjoy creating new recipes. Unless you are only drinking a single serving of fruit juice (which is typically 4 ounces), limit your fruit juice intake. Fruit juice has a high sugar content and can cause your blood sugar level to spike. Try to limit fruit to a 1:4 ratio of fruit juice to vegetable juice. You may want to start off with sweeter juices but have a single serving.

Main Ingredient - Base

Choosing produce that contains a high liquid content can help you cut costs and make for more delicious juices.

Adding juices with high water content helps flush your system and makes your juices flavorful, light, and gentler for detoxing. The following produce recommendations are all low in fat, sodium, and calories. They also do not have any cholesterol. (Due to its' high sugar content, limit fruit juice to a 1:4 ratio when combining it with vegetable juice.)

Cucumber

Cucumbers are a favorite vegetable to use as each individual cucumber yields a high amount of liquid.

- Benefits: Cucumbers have a beneficial amount of vitamin K, sulfur, potassium, and manganese. Due to their rejuvenating properties, they are great for the skin, hair, and nails.

Celery

Celery is great for adding a bit of saltiness to your juice, making it savory.

- Benefits: Celery has a slightly salty taste while being low in sodium. It contains zeaxanthin and lutein which could potentially minimize the risk of eye disease. Celery also assists with high blood pressure and rheumatoid arthritis. In addition, it helps the body cool down and reduces one's cravings for sweets.

Carrots

Carrots are an excellent way to sweeten your vegetable juice.

- Benefits: Carrots contain vitamin A and carotenoids including alpha and beta-carotene. They are beneficial to eye and bone health and assist in absorbing free radicals. Carrots may also aid in cancer prevention of the stomach, mouth, and lungs.

Apples - Green and Fuji

Apples are an excellent fruit that yields a high amount of juice in addition to sweetening other juices. (Note - apples create a lot of foam.)

- Benefits: Apples have an excellent source of pectin, potassium, and vitamin C. They have phytochemicals which can aid in averting diseases such as heart disease, diabetes, high cholesterol, and cancer. Apples help remove toxins from the body and assist in flushing out the kidneys.

Pineapples

Pineapples are another great fruit to sweeten your juice and change the flavor.

- Benefits: Pineapples are a useful source of vitamin C. They contain bromelain, an enzyme that aids in digestion and can assist with indigestion and assists with blood clots.

Oranges

Oranges have a detoxing effect. Pair them with grapefruit, lemon, and ginger for a great system flush.

- Benefits: Oranges contain vitamin C which boosts the immune system. They are an excellent source of phytochemicals that help with inflammation and may hinder cancer.

Water

Use filtered or distilled water and add to taste.

- Benefits: Water flushes the system. It stretches your juice to make more ounces. Water dilutes juices that may otherwise be too potent for your body which can result in increased detox systems. It can also make juices more palatable.

Other Great Produce

Below is a short list of produce to use. Reference the "Shopping List" section for a more thorough list.

Leafy greens

Green juices have an excellent cleansing effect. Use leafy greens such as kale, spinach, chard, dandelion greens, cabbage, arugula, and beet greens.

Vegetables

Sweet potato, radish, beets, and bell pepper (all colors).

Fruit

Grapes, grapefruit, pomegranate, watermelon, cantaloupe, and honeydew.

Herbs and Spices

Cayenne is an excellent spice. It is known to be anti-bacterial and stimulate acid in the stomach.

Cilantro is known for removing metal from the body. It can assist in preventing inflammation. It is also a good source of phytochemicals such as beta-carotene, rutin, and apigenin.

Parsley has antioxidants such as lutein and quercetin which support eye health. It also has vitamins A, C, and K.

Add-Ons

Lemons are an excellent diuretic and help remove toxins from the body.

Ginger assists with circulation opens your sinuses and helps relieve nausea. Also, it may help with rheumatoid arthritis.

Seaweed, such as blue-green algae, spirulina, and dulse, can contribute iodine to your diet and can benefit an underactive thyroid.

Sea salt contains trace minerals, such as magnesium, potassium, and calcium, which are beneficial to your system.

Drink the Rainbow

Why Should You Drink Colorful Produce?

Juice in colors to ensure that you are receiving a balance of nutrients. Specific colors generally have a higher concentration of a specific nutrient. When you think of carrots, sweet potato, and cantaloupe, what nutrient comes to mind? You most likely thought of beta-carotene.

When completing an extended juice fast, try to incorporate each of the colors in your diet through the day. Below is a quick, high-level list of what the following colors can do for your body.

Red

- Benefits: Red foods are known for containing betacyanins which help in conditions such as cancer. Red foods are also known for having lycopene. Lycopene is beneficial to the prostate gland and the lungs. Lycopene has been shown to avert conditions such as heart disease, cataracts, and breast cancer.

- Examples: Great red foods for juicing are beets, tomatoes, red bell pepper, cranberries, pomegranate seeds, watermelon.

White

- Benefits: Allicin, in garlic and onions, is both antifungal and antibacterial. It helps ward off infection.

- Examples: Garlic, onion, ginger.

Yellow/Orange

- Benefits: Yellow and orange foods are known for having carotenoid compounds. This colorful produce contain compounds such as lutein and zeaxanthin. Orange is also known for beta-carotene and lycopene. The color of carotenoids can range from yellow to a bright red or orange. The deeper the color orange, the more concentrated the compound. This compound has been found to be beneficial to eyesight. It has also been found to minimize the risk of cancers such as prostate, esophagus, bladder, and colon cancer.

- Examples: Yellow foods include lemons, pineapple, grapefruit, oranges, and yellow bell peppers. Beautiful juices can be created by orange foods such as orange bell pepper, orange beets, carrots, butternut squash, and cantaloupe.

Blue/Purple

- Benefits: Blue and purple foods are known for containing antioxidants which provide protection from free radicals.

- Examples: purple or red cabbage, purple kale.

Green

- Benefits: Mom always said to eat your greens. She was right. Green produce incorporates all of the benefits of each color. Green vegetables are known for chlorophyll. They also have antioxidants and phytonutrients. While juicing, including leafy greens and green vegetables daily is essential.

- Examples: A few green foods are spinach, kale, chard, collards, celery, cucumber, beet greens, dandelion greens, arugula, romaine lettuce, cabbage, green pepper, and herbs such as parsley and cilantro.

Supplements

Supplements help minimize the detox symptoms, add nutritional value to the fast, and help remove metal and toxins from the body. Although they are optional, you may find adding one or two of these will help you achieve your desired results.

Bee Pollen

Bee pollen contains almost all the nutrients humans need. It improves energy, reduces cravings, and helps prevent everyday ailments.

Cascara Sagrada

Cascara Sagrada generally comes in capsule form. This herbal remedy is generally used as a laxative and will assist you in eliminating waste.

Coconut Oil

Your skin is your body's largest organ. Coconut oil is beneficial both externally and internally. Use coconut oil as an alternative to skin care products that have chemicals and additives. When ingested, it aids in weight loss, increased energy and memory, and more.

Smooth Move

Smooth Move is a tea that assists with elimination. It contains senna leaf and other herbs that are known for their laxative effects. Drink this tea before bed.

Salt Water Flush

Salt Water Flush is a process that also has a laxative effect. When completed correctly, the salt is flushed from your system.

Green Powder

Green powders are a popular choice for juice fasts. They provide vital minerals and nutrients. They are not considered a supplement but a whole food. A quality green powder has vegetables, pre- and probiotics, digestive enzymes, sea vegetables, and other beneficial additives.

MSM

MSM is methylsulfonylmethane also known as glucosamine MSM. During weight loss, it is an excellent supplement for joints and inflammation. It assists with collagen and helps repairs your skin tone and elasticity.

Sesame Oil

Sesame oil is a warming moisturizer for your skin. It is naturally antibacterial and antiviral. It can help with inflammation and has been used to assist in reversing common ailments.

Spirulina

Spirulina is a blue-green algae known for eliminating heavy metals from the body, assisting with weight loss and sinus issues, and boosting energy. It also packs a right amount of protein.

Zeolite

Zeolite is available in liquid or powder form. It is an absorbent known to pull heavy metal and toxins such as aluminum from the body.

The Fast

Pre-Fast

To be successful in your fast, set yourself up to succeed. The following tips will help you begin your fast in a safe way and can ease anxiety about the experience.

Foods to Avoid

It is essential to prepare your body for fasting. Easing into the fast will prevent your body from attempting to detox too fast thus easing reactions such as bloating, hives, headaches, and even flu-like symptoms.

I recommend doing a variation of the Elimination Diet and the Mucusless Diet by Professor Arnold Ehret, before a juice fast. This is the process of removing common allergens and mucus forming foods from your diet such as corn, potatoes, and dairy.

When selecting meals, try to pick foods other than those listed below and/or do not have these ingredients listed in the first five on the label. Do not get overwhelmed. Begin by minimizing. For example, if you are completing a 7-day fast, three days before, if you generally drink 2 cups of coffee, only drink 1. Then, two days before, drink a ½ cup and one day before drink a ¼ cup or no coffee at all.

Foods to eliminate:

Corn

Potatoes

Gluten/Wheat

Yeast

Dairy

Peanuts

Eggs

Meat

Caffeine

Processed and Refined Carbohydrates and Sugar

High Corn Fructose Syrup

Hydrogenated (Trans) Fats

Canned, Processed, Packaged, Junk, or Fast Foods

Alcohol

Foods high in sodium

Fried Foods

Salt

Set Your Intentions

Setting your intentions can be one of the most influential things you do on a fast. When you set your intentions, make sure they are personal, inspiring, and meaningful to you. For example: to have a vibrant long life for your children, to connect more spiritually, to lose weight to fit into your dream wedding dress.

When you set your intentions on something that is meaningful, if you begin to have second thoughts, you can refer to your reasons and remember why it is essential to stay on track.

When I set intentions on my juice fast and maintaining a high raw foods diet, it was for preventative maintenance. I have a history of obesity, diabetes, hypertension, and cancer that run in my family. I wanted to make sure that I was not taking medication when I reached 40. I knew that my longevity, health, and happiness were dependent upon the success of me changing my diet and lifestyle.

I now consider and understand the quote "Food is the best form of medicine or your slowest poison" by Ann Wigmore. Given a chance, our bodies can heal and repair themselves on a daily basis.

Support System

Research shows that people are more likely to be successful if they think about their goals. The rate of success increases if you write down your goals. There is another increase if you write <u>and</u> speak your goals out loud. There is yet another increase if you share your goals. Lastly, having an accountability partner that is nonjudgmental and supportive can make all the difference in your success.

Having a sense of community is essential. Consider joining social communities that focus on juice fasting, look for local meet-up groups, and consider fasting with friends. If you decide to do a 7-day fast, maybe you can get a couple of friends that will offset your fast with a pair of 3-day fasts.

When I completed my 60-day fast, I participated in a Facebook group that had access to peer health coaches whom themselves were doing detoxes during my fast. That was incredible to know that someone else was in it with me, even if their fast was only for 3 days. The coaches were my biggest cheerleaders. They checked in on me regularly, they asked questions, and they gave me kudos that helped to push me forward.

Be careful of people that may add unneeded stress. If you know of friends and family that may not be supportive, you can limit what you share with them. I have people that inadvertently made me feel awkward or dampened my spirits. I received feedback such as I couldn't possibly do that; Is that safe, what about your protein and calcium, don't you need fiber, can I juice burger and fries, well while you are doing that I'm going to eat this donut, aren't you sure you don't want a little of my food. For them, it may have been in good spirits. However, it was not encouraging to me, and it was a distraction from my end goal.

If I had not been strong, I could have easily been swayed from meeting my goals. Because you are sharing your thoughts on food without realizing it, people naturally want to share what they are eating for dinner, how they binged on ice cream this weekend, or talk about the barbecue they have coming up. It can be disheartening and make you feel like you are on an island all alone.

Share with those that may give you helpful juicing recipes and tips, someone that may want to complete one day of fasting with you, someone that may be interested and will help you research, or someone who will just check in on you and encourage you if you need it.

The Fast

Preparation is key

Before the fast, find juice recipes that interest you. Find out what appliances and tools you need, make your shopping list, and go shopping.

When preparing produce for juicing, make sure you wash it thoroughly. Rinse fruit with skin, even if you are not using the skin, like lemons, grapefruit, and pineapples. Rinsing them will keep dirt and bacteria from contaminating the flesh of the produce when you cut through it.

Prepare your juice, place it in airtight containers, and refrigerate it if you decide to juice once and drink throughout the day.

Shortcuts: Pre-Prep, Juice Bars

I have had several successful 7-14 day fasts where I purchased juice. Research juice bars and natural food stores near you. Several juice bars provide unpasteurized juice along with detox packages that can help cut costs. Some natural food stores will allow you to pick your fresh fruit and vegetables from their produce section and then make and bottle your juice for free or nominal amount.

If you are in a pinch and unable to get fresh juice, purchase juice that is either cold-pressed, flash-pasteurized, or a local store's variety. Juice from concentrate is not recommended due to its low nutritional value and possible additives. Coconut water and Master Cleanse are my favorite go-to when I don't have time to shop. See the "Eating on the Go" section for more details.

Sample Day

<u>*Morning*</u>

Journaling

Lemon Water with upgrades 16 ounces

Meditation Yoga Walk

Alkaline Juice 20 – 32 ounces

<u>*Mid-Morning*</u>

Basic Juice 20 – 32 ounces

<u>*Afternoon*</u>

Basic/Alkaline Juice 20 – 32 ounces

<u>*Evening*</u>

Basic/Alkaline Juice (opt) 20 – 32 ounces

Rebounding Walk

<u>*Late Night*</u>

Alkaline Juice- last meal before bedtime 20 – 32 ounces (optional)

Journaling and writing notes of gratitude

Breaking the Fast

Breaking your fast, post-detox, is one of the most critical parts of the fast. If you are doing a countdown to fast completion, include the post days in your program. Including the days will mentally prepare you for the actual end of the detox program. Trust me when I say that you will be excited about breaking your fast. Prunes, apples, fruit with high water content, and simple salads will taste divine. When you are new to the process, mainly if you regularly consume a Standard American Diet, you may be excited about incorporating other foods immediately and become overzealous. If you begin knowing that it is going to take an additional 1-3 days to get back to your diet, it will help you be mentally prepared for those days and know that the fast is not over until after the post-detox is complete.

Introducing Food Back Into Your Diet

Incorporate foods into your diet slowly. Your organs have taken a break from digestion and need to wake up gradually. Eating heavy foods too soon can leave you feeling bloated and lock up your system. Depending on the length of the fast, you can begin introducing foods in this order: foods that digest the fastest, high water content fruit and vegetables, and then denser foods.

If you only replaced breakfast with juice, then you can have a nice healthy lunch with no concern. If you completed a 1-day fast, breaking the fast with fruit or a smoothie in the morning and a nice healthy meal later is acceptable. If you end a 3-day fast, on your fourth day, you may want to go with a raw food diet for the entire fourth day to help your body begin to digest whole food again. For a 7-day or longer fast, you will want to take three days or longer to transition out of the fast.

Do not sabotage your efforts once the fast is complete. It took a lot of discipline to complete your goal. Refer back to your intentions to remember why you did the detox in the first place. Why did you decide to accomplish this goal? How do your intentions impact your after-fasting goals? Will you cut back on sugar? Will you switch to lean cuts of meat? Will you slow down on eating fried food?

Where you can, plan out your next steps ahead of time. If you can plan out your new diet and lifestyle before beginning the juice fast, it will help you get mentally prepared, and then you will not have to think about tempting foods while going through the fast.

After my 60-day fast, I wanted to continue on my journey without dairy and meat for as long as it resonated with my body. I was able to complete the detox plan and begin my journey successfully without any temptation or feelings of deprivation. I was mentally prepared and ready for my new lifestyle.

What do you want to accomplish with your diet and lifestyle? Do you want to reverse a common ailment? Is it for preventative maintenance? Is it for longevity or the fountain of youth? Once you know what you want to accomplish, you can sit down with your doctor or naturopath to create a diet and regimen that works for you. Where you can look for a meal plan that you can make into a permanent lifestyle.

Research books and resources on the internet. Remember, however, that the information written does not know your unique health history and a lot of it is contradictory. Use your intuition and learn who the respected health leaders are that get the results you want.

If you are looking for holistic methods for curing eczema, you may want to talk with someone that healed themselves with natural ingredients. Find someone that has a track record of working with people with the condition you want to reverse. Ask for referrals and review testimonials.

I had the opportunity to volunteer at the Living Foods Institute for a year. I was able to witness firsthand people's results on a raw foods diet versus reading about it online and questioning the legitimacy.

Raw Foods Diet

The Raw Foods Diet is an excellent way to transition out of a juice fast. The foods on this plan encourage continued detox and help provide the nutrients necessary for the body to continue to heal and operate optimally.

Wikipedia Definition of Raw Foodism and Raw Foodist

Raw Foodism is a lifestyle promoting the consumption of uncooked, unprocessed, and often organic foods as a large percentage of the diet. Depending on the type of lifestyle and results desired, raw food diets may include a selection of raw fruits, vegetables, nuts, seeds (including sprouted whole grains), eggs, fish, meat, and unpasteurized dairy products (such as raw milk, cheese, and yogurt).

A raw foodist is a person who consumes primarily raw food, or all raw food, depending on how strict the diet is. Raw foodists typically believe that the higher the percentage of raw food in the diet, the higher the health benefits. Members of the raw food community claim that raw food encourages weight loss and prevents and/or heals many forms of sickness and many chronic diseases.

What is a Raw Foodist?

A raw foodist is a person whose diet is made up of 75% or more of raw foods.

Raw foodists believe that the maximum benefits are seen at 100% raw food intake.

What are Raw Foods?

Raw foods are living foods that have living enzymes.

Enzymes are no longer present in food prepared at a range of 105-116 degrees.

Foods that have been cooked, processed, and/or pasteurized over 115 degrees are not raw.

If it does not state on the label that it is raw or living, it may not be raw.

Raw foods may include vegetables, cultured vegetables, sea vegetables, fruit, seeds, sprouted grains, and sprouted nuts.

Detox Tools

Skin Brushing

Skin brushing is an easy way to help you detox. It helps with circulation, your lymph nodes, remove dead skin cells from the body and helps release trapped impurities. To skin brush, you typically hold the brush firmly in your hand and stroke your skin toward your heart. Be careful to avoid areas that may be sensitive to the brushing. For example, brush from ankle to knee, knee to hip, wrist to elbow, and elbow to shoulder. Stroke each area approximately ten times. Upon completion, take a refreshing shower or a contrast shower.

Contrast Shower

A contrast shower is good for detoxing as well. A contrast shower is an act of turning on the hot water to as hot as you can stand it without burning yourself, for a preset amount of time, then turning the water to as cold as you can stand it for that same amount of time and then repeating. When the water is hot, it dilates your blood vessels, and blood rushes to your skin increasing your circulation. When the water is cold, the blood vessels constrict which decreases circulation. This process helps circulate your blood, helps with sore muscles, and does wonders for your skin.

Tongue Scraping

Your tongue is one of the most prominent mirrors of what is happening in your body. When you are going through detox, your tongue will naturally develop a coat of film. These are the impurities that are coming from your body to the surface of your tongue. Purchase a tongue scraper and scrape your tongue at least twice a day. This will help remove the film and freshen your breath.

Enema Kit

Enemas help flush out your lower colon and remove toxins. It is recommended to do an enema upon waking daily for the first week or so when juice fasting. When completing a fast, your body is attempting to eliminate as many toxins as possible. Enemas help to remove toxins and prevent these impurities from being reabsorbed into your organs and tissue.

Oil Pulling

Oil pulling has existed for ages and is primarily used in Ayurvedic medicine. It is useful for pulling out toxins through your tongue and gums. The process begins with placing 1-2 tablespoons of oil (such as coconut oil, olive oil, or sesame oil) in your mouth and swishing it gently between your teeth and through your mouth for 10-20 minutes.

Colonics

A colonic (also known as hydrocolonic, colon cleansing, colonic irrigation) is the act of having filtered water flush toxins and impacted fecal matter from your colon and intestines. The process is more thorough than an enema as it can flush out from deeper within your system. Your intestines can have years of fecal matter impacted inside. After a series of colonics, people tend to feel lighter physically and mentally, have better skin, and much more.

Tips and Tricks

Be Prepared

Mentally and physically, be prepared. Have all the resources and supplements you need in advance.

Physically Prepared

Plan how you will get your juice, whether buying it pre-bottled or preparing it yourself.

Purchasing juice from the store? Make sure the flavors you wish to purchase are available, and research bundles like Buy 10 Get 1 Free. Will the store be closed for the holiday? Are there particular events that may prevent you from getting to the store? Do you need to pre-purchase packages?

Juicing on your own? Do you have the juicer you intend to use? Do you have your other supplies: mason jars, glass straws, tongue scraper, etc.? Do you have the supplements that you want on this journey? Get all the tools and resources you need weeks ahead of time.

Research in advance. Please do not wait until the day of to find out if ginger is okay to juice if you are taking medication. Figure out what produce you want to avoid and what fruit and vegetables you want to incorporate for specific benefits. For instance, you may want to incorporate blue-green algae if you have an underactive thyroid or cucumbers for glowing skin.

Will you run to your favorite fast-food restaurant the day before the juice fast? Eating such food will increase your risk of detox symptoms. You can have inflammation, intense headaches, aches, and pains in places you did not know existed as a result.

Make sure you are being smart and using the Elimination Diet when beginning a fast. Someone following a vegan whole foods diet might be able to start a detox immediately. However, a person that regularly has heavy starches, dairy, meat, and caffeine will want to transition to detox over one to three weeks before an extended fast.

Mentally Prepared

Do you have the journal you want to use? Have you chosen the type of spiritual connection you want to do? Do you own any meditation music? Do you know what parks you want to visit? What other mini vacations can you go on physically <u>and</u> mentally?

Most of juicing is a mental process. We are conditioned to live to eat versus eating to live. We want to eat what we want to eat when we want to eat it. Addictions to food do not make it easier. What will you do when you have a craving? What happens when you have that birthday party to attend? What about when you just want something to chew? Any number of roadblocks may present themselves. Being mentally prepared by knowing how you will address these situations is essential.

Be clear on the length of your entire detox process. People tend to think the juice fast starts the day you begin drinking juice. In essence, it begins anywhere from one to seven days before with the pre-detox, depending on the length of the fast and your current diet and lifestyle. Also, take into consideration that the post-fast can extend up to a week after you finish juicing.

Journaling

Journaling is an excellent way to track your progress and your feelings throughout the journey. You will be able to see what foods resonate with your body and help you feel your best or, conversely, lower your energy. As you become in tune with your body, you may be able to recognize foods that are causing ailments such as inflammation, joint pain, and more. Some produce may make you feel a little more lethargic. Some foods will give you a boost of energy.

Another thing to take note of is a potential emotional detox. You may experience a feeling of sadness or lethargy for reasons unknown or reliving something that you have not thought of in years. This is absolutely normal. It is a process. This is another reason journaling and "me time" is essential.

It would be great if you write upon rising and just before bed.

Affirmations

Affirmations are one of your most powerful and inspirational tools in your toolbox. Affirmations are a series of positive words or phrases that can be repeated several times. These words generally encourage self-empowerment and give a person the "I can" attitude. A few affirmations that may sound familiar to you are listed below.

"I think I can, I think I can," said by The Little Engine that Could

"I think, therefore I am," by Rene Descartes

Affirmations are an underutilized tool in our society. If you are new to affirmations, I greatly recommend the book "You can Heal Your Life" by Louise L Hay.

Below a few quotes or affirmations that may resonate with you:

- I am love

- I am beautiful

- I am life

- I am healthy and receive the life force I need to have a vibrant and healthy body

- I am worth this beautiful journey

- I will continue this journey with ease

Connect with Nature

When I was completing my fast, I began to connect more with nature. I wanted to open all the blinds in the house. I wanted to see the sunshine. I wanted to be out at the park, on the grass and be close to nature. Being in nature has many healing qualities. It not only rejuvenates the soul but allows you to get movement and exercise as well. If you have the opportunity, kick off your shoes and take a nice barefoot walk in the grass.

Can I Buy Juice?

Absolutely. Some options can minimize your time in the kitchen. Please note that you will pay for the convenience. However, depending on your budget and time, it can be beneficial. See the "Eating on the Go" section for more information.

Will I Be Hungry?

You should not be starving while juicing. Find out what works for you. Some people drink a gallon by drinking 8 ounces every hour until they are finished drinking for the day. Some people mimic their mealtimes: 20-32 ounces for breakfast, lunch, snack, and dinner. During the fast, you should continue to drink water. You can drink up to a gallon of juice or more if needed. If you are hungry, drink more juice.

How Long Does the Juice Keep?

It is best to ingest juice after it has been extracted. However, depending on the type of juicer you use and how you package your juice, it can keep up to 3 days. Try to fill the juice to the rim to keep air from being in your jar. If you need to, put the juice in the freezer until the next morning.

Bear in mind that different produce oxidizes at various rates. Celery tends to maintain its taste while the taste of other produce can begin to disappear. If your juice starts to taste fermented or feels fizzy on your tongue, it is time to discard it.

Protein and Calcium

Most produce contains protein and calcium. If you are completing a short fast, one or two days of limited amounts of both will not be a cause for concern. Spinach and other leafy greens are an excellent source of both. There was a reason Popeye made us want to eat our spinach. You can incorporate powders such as spirulina or chlorella, and other super green powders, to supplement your juices.

Fiber and Elimination

Your bowels contain years of impacted fecal matter. It is ordinary and necessary to eliminate waste during your fast. It is essential to remove the toxins from your body to prevent them from reabsorbing in your cells, organs, and tissue.

Remember, as you are juicing, your body is removing as many toxins as it can. If it cannot eliminate them through urination and bowel movement, it will try to remove the toxins in other ways. This can cause hives, boils, and other physical ailments. Make sure you are eliminating on a regular basis and consider cleansing your colon with an enema kit or receiving a colonic. I chose to use cascara sagrada or Smooth Move Tea, and I received colonics at least twice a week. During my extended fast, I did enemas every day.

Eating on the Go
Traveling and Restaurants

Are you too busy to prepare? Is life getting in the way? When I first began juicing regularly, I started planning out my health goals for the year. I knew I wanted to do quarterly detoxes, whether through juicing or food. As I looked at my calendar, I became distraught. My calendar was full of triathlon training, a full-time job, facilitating workshops and, my biggest concern, several trips. I began to wonder if it was a smart to plan an extended juice fast while traveling. Then I thought about how I continued my 60-day juice fast in 2012 even while traveling for a few days across the U.S.

I have juice fasted regularly over the past several years. I knew there would not be a perfect time. However, I knew I could complete a fast even with the travel I had planned and you can too.

Below are easy steps to complete a juice fast while traveling or at home successfully.

Decide if you are juicing yourself or if you will find local juice at your destination. This will help you plan what to bring during your fast. It will also help you decide what you need to search for on the internet. Search for the closest grocery stores, local juice bars, farmers' markets, raw vegan restaurants, and similar places.

Call those places to ensure they are open and ask any questions, including about possible delivery service. You may even want to track the distance between these locations to where you are staying. Will you be able to walk there? Can you get there on a bus or train? If so, how much will it cost? You may pay more than you usually would for your juices.

Always have a standby juice ready. Juicing while on a flight. Many airports have juice bars. A lot of restaurants prepare freshly squeezed juice. Several kiosks have pasteurized juice and unpasteurized juice that you can carry with you to your destination.

The Master Cleanse is the most accessible juice to make on the fly. In your carry-on bag, take plenty of lemons, cayenne pepper, and maple syrup/raw agave. This standby juice can be used throughout the trip if you choose. When I was completing my 60-day juice fast, I made my juice right on the plane. When I got to the airport and past security, I purchased a couple of bottles of water and was able to make my juice before I boarded the plane. Consider coconut water as an option.

Juicing at your destination. This is where all of your pre-work comes in handy. You will want to make a trip to the market or grocery store. You will also want to consider if your destination has a juicer that you can use if there is a refrigerator available, do you need to bring mason jars, and other concerns.

Stores now sell small juicers that are portable and can be put in luggage. I have a friend that travels with her juicer. Once she arrives at her destination, she purchases produce, and voila, she juices in her hotel room.

Find juice at your destination. If you are going to a major city, it's easy to find juice at local juice bars, farmers markets, raw vegan restaurants, and similar places. When I was in Long Island, California, I was able to take a taxi to a local juice bar. I bought enough juice for two days. Due to the amount of juice I purchased, the juice bar not only gave me an extra juice for free, but they also gave me a free juice for my taxi driver!

Lastly, remember to surround yourself with supportive family and friends. Share your expectations and wishes as it pertains to your juice fast with each other. Juice fasts can require more trips and attention that may change travel plans. Having their commitment ahead of time can be a great help.

By planning ahead, completing a juice fast while traveling can be accomplished with ease. Do not overthink it. You already have the discipline to finish a juice fast. Find the fastest and easiest way to get the juice you need and enjoy your trip!

I'm So Over This Juice!

Save your favorite juice for the difficult times. There may be a point during your juice fast that you do not want to look at or smell juice anymore. Save your favorite or most decadent juices for such times. Make a broth that has sea salt that you usually do not add or with produce that adds lots of delicious flavors but may be more expensive to purchase.

Change it up. Try freezing your favorite treat juice into a popsicle. Keep these tips in your back pocket. This is an excellent way to revitalize your fast and help you look forward to tasty treats.

Coconut Oil - It is okay to have one tablespoon of coconut oil every other day or so. I suggest putting the oil in the refrigerator or freezer until it is solid and then biting into it to elevate that sensation of biting.

Bee Pollen - Another supplement you can have daily is bee pollen. Take one tablespoon and chew on it. It will dissolve in your mouth or in juice.

Also, refer back to your intentions. Why are you completing this fast? Remember that you can do it! You are worth it!

Pasteurized and Conventional Store Bought Juices

Let's discuss freshly pressed versus pasteurized. If you can, freshly juice your produce for consumption. However, if you only have access to conventional 100% juice, do not let that stop you from your fast. Coconut water and detox juices that you can be purchased at natural food stores or juice bars are excellent. Make sure they are 100% juice and try to buy local pasteurized versions instead of the popular juice brands. Look for words such as cold-pressed where possible. I successfully completed a 2-day detox with juices that I bought at a major natural food store.

Additional Things to Consider

While you are juice fasting, continue to drink plenty of water. Many times when you're drinking nearly a gallon of juice, you may not feel like you need to drink water. However, your body is removing and flushing out toxins at a rapid pace. Water will aid in removing those toxins from your system.

Where you can, choose high-quality produce while it is in season. Organic fresh fruit and vegetables are ideal. If you are unable to access all organic, where you can, shop from the "Dirty Dozen" and "Clean 10" lists. For example, purchase organic leafy green vegetables or conventional carrots and then peel the skin.

If you are unable to get organic, please do not let that stop you. You can still receive many benefits from juicing unconventional juice.

Since you are cleansing, you might as well bump it up a notch! Consider doing a liver, spleen, and gallbladder juice cleanse while you are fasting. Try one of the various cleanses that assist with specific organs. Do a little research to find what works for you.

Shopping Guide

Juice Fasting Shopping List

When I decided to fast, it was essential to have some basic items to be successful. Here are a few items you may select. Please note, you want to buy local, in season, and organic as much as possible. To save money, buy in bulk or on sale where you can. My local farmers market gives a discount for buying the full box of produce. My local natural food grocery store gives a 10% discount when you buy the full box. I have taken advantage of these opportunities numerous times. Do not overwhelm yourself.

BARE NECESSITIES

Vegetables - Remember, when shopping for green vegetables, the greener the better. For other vegetables, look for deep vibrant color! The more colorful your diet, the more well-rounded your nutrition. Variety is key in juicing. Make it a habit of trying something different.

Leafy Greens - Do not overlook the following green vegetables:

Collard Green Leaf

Kale (curly and dinosaur)

Parsley (all types)

Bok Choy

Spinach

Dandelion Greens

Beet Greens

Basil

Fruit - Fruit is abundant. Pick any juicy fruit that you like. Keep in mind that fruit will only make up about a quarter of your daily intake.

When possible, pick fruit with seeds. Fruit without seeds are not produced by nature and have less nutritional value. The more seeds it has, the less it has been genetically altered.

Apples

Oranges

Pineapple

Cranberry

Pomegranate

Tomato

Grapes

Blood Orange

Muscadine

Sea Vegetables - Sea vegetables are ideal for iodine and trace minerals.

Wakame

Dulse

Drinks/Smoothies

Tea (Yerba Mate, herbal)

Water

Thai/Green Coconuts

Fresh Juices

Fresh Herbs/Spices/Condiments

Fresh Squeezed Lemon/Lime Juice

Raw Apple Cider Vinegar

Olive Oil (cold or first-pressed)

Ginger

High-Quality Sea Salt

Cayenne Pepper

Superfoods

Flaxseed Oil

Bee Pollen

Coconut Oil

Supplements

Green Powders

Smooth Move Tea

MSM Powder

Zeolite

Body

Sesame Oil

Coconut Oil

Enema Kit

Recipe Combinations

I frequently get asked what I put in my juice. It changes so often because I use a quick rule of thumb. I use 5 ingredients or less which includes; a base, a leafy green vegetable, one or two other fruit or vegetables of choice and an upgrade. More than that can either get overwhelming or pricy. Keep it simple. Find two recipe overviews below.

Regular Recipes

Choose a base: carrot, apple, or pineapple 2-8 oz

Add one leafy green vegetable (optional) 1 oz

Add two or three other fruits or vegetables 10-12 oz

Upgrade: add lemon, ginger, cayenne, herbs, and/or spices

Green Recipes – Low Glycemic

Choose a base: cucumber, celery, carrot, or water 8-10 oz

Add one leafy green vegetable (optional) 2 oz

Add one or two other green vegetables 2-8 oz

Upgrade: add lemon, ginger, cayenne, herbs, and/or spices

3- Day Regular Plan

Grocery List for Regular 3-Day Plan

Salad, enough for Pre and Post Detox
4 oz Veggie Kraut
4 TB Ground Flax
4 Orange
11 Lemon (Get more to add for taste)
2 Lime
1 Large Grapefruit
25 Cucumber (You may want to get extra to add more liquid)
16 Large Zucchini
4 Large Beets
11 Apple (You may want to get extra to add more liquid)
1-2 Bunches of Kale
39 Celery Stalks (You may want to get extra to add more liquid)
1 Bunch of Chard
1-2 Bunches of Parsley
1 Bunch of Cilantro
1 Bunch of Dill
Cumin
Cayenne (Optional)
Turmeric (Optional)

3-Day Regular Juices Menu

Pre-Detox

Salad / 2 oz. Veggie Kraut / 2TB Ground Flax

3-Day Menu

Day 1

Juice 1 – 4 Orange / 2 Lemon / 2 Lime / 1 Grapefruit

Juice 2 – 3 Cucumber / 1 Beet / 1 Lemon / 1 Apple

Juice 3 – 3 Cucumber / 2 Leaves of Kale / 4 Celery Stalks / 1 Apple/ Lemon to taste

Juice 4 - 3 Cucumber/ 2 Leaves of Kale / 5 Celery Stalks / 2 Leaves of Chard / 7 sprigs of Parsley / Lemon to taste

Day 2

Juice 1 – 2 Chard / 5 Celery Stalks / 3 Cucumber / 1 Apple/ 1 Lemon

Juice 2 – 2 Apple / 2 Beet / 1 Lemon / 6-8 Celery Stalks / 5 sprigs of Parsley

Juice 3 – 2 Cucumber / 7 sprigs of Cilantro / 4 Celery Stalks / 2-3 Apples / 1 Lemon

Juice 4 (broth) – 6-8 Zucchini / 7 sprigs of Dill / 4 Celery Stalks / Cumin to taste

Day 3

Juice 1 – 5 Celery Stalks / 3 Cucumber / 1 Lemon

Juice 2 - 4 Cucumber / 1 Beet / 1 Lemon / 2 Apple

Juice 3 - 3 Cucumber / 2 Leaves of Kale / 4 Celery Stalks / 1 Apple/ Lemon to taste

Juice 4 (broth) – 6-8 Zucchini / 7 sprigs of Dill / 4 sprigs of Parsley / 3 leaves of Kale / Cumin to taste

Note- Ounces varies depending on the size of the produce and the type of juicer you have. Adding more cucumber and/or celery will help to add more liquid to your juice.

Post-Detox

Salad / 2 oz. Veggie Kraut / 2 TB Ground Flax

3-DAY GREEN JUICE MENU

Grocery List for Regular 3-Day Plan
Salad, enough for Pre and Post Detox
4 oz Veggie Kraut
4 TB Ground Flax
8 Lemon (Get more to add for taste)
Lime (Optional for taste)
26 Large Cucumber (You may want to get extra to add more liquid)
28 Large Zucchini
 Apple (Optional, use sparingly)
3 Large Bunches of Kale
5 Bunches of Celery (You may want to get extra to add more liquid)
1 Bunch of Chard
1 Bunch of Spinach
1 Head of Romaine
1 Bunch of Parsley
1 Bunch of Dill
Cumin
Cayenne (Optional)
Turmeric (Optional)

Pre-Detox
Salad / 2 oz Veggie Kraut / 2 TB Ground Flax

3-Day Menu
Day 1

Juice 1 - 4 Cucumber / 2 Leaves of Kale / 4 Celery Stalks / Handful of Spinach leaves / Lemon to taste

Juice 2 - 5 Celery / 3 Cucumber / 1 Lemon

Juice 3 - 4 Cucumber / 2 Leaves of Kale / 4 Celery Stalks / Lemon to taste

Juice 4 (broth) – 6-8 Zucchini / 7 sprigs of Dill / 4 Celery Stalks / Cumin to taste

Day 2

Juice 1 - 2 Chard / 5 Celery Stalks / 4 Cucumber / 1 Lemon

Juice 2 - 4 Cucumber / 2 Leaves of Kale / 5 Celery Stalks / 2 Leaves of Chard / 7 sprigs of Parsley / Lemon to taste

Juice 3 - 4 Cucumber / 2 Leaves of Kale / 4 Celery Stalks / Lemon to taste

Juice 4 (broth) – 6-8 Zucchini / 7 sprigs of Dill / 4 sprigs of Parsley / 3 leaves of Kale / Cumin to taste

Day 3

Juice 1 - 5 Celery Stalks / 3 Cucumber / 1 Lemon / Handful of Spinach Leaves

Juice 2 - 5 Celery Stalks / 1 Lemon / 6-8 leaves of Romaine

Juice 3 - 4 Zucchini / 7 sprigs of Dill / 5 Celery Stalks

Juice 4 (broth) – 6-8 Zucchini / 7 sprigs of Dill / 3 leaves of Kale / Cumin to taste

Post-Detox

Salad / 2 oz Veggie Kraut / 2 TB Ground Flax

Note- Ounces varies depending on the size of the produce and the type of juicer you have. Adding more cucumber and/or celery will help to add more liquid to your juice.

Getting Ready

Try to complete this section 1-2 two weeks prior to your fast.

What are your intentions for this juice fast? (for detox, mental clarity, jump start weight loss or a diet regimen)

Let's go deeper. Answer why again. (why is detox important to you, why do you really want to lose weight?)

No really, I need you to dig deeper, WHY? What's in it for you, for your family and friends, for you impact with those around you?

Do you have a support system? Who and what does that support system look like to you?

Are they willing to help you when you have questions or if you begin to have doubts?

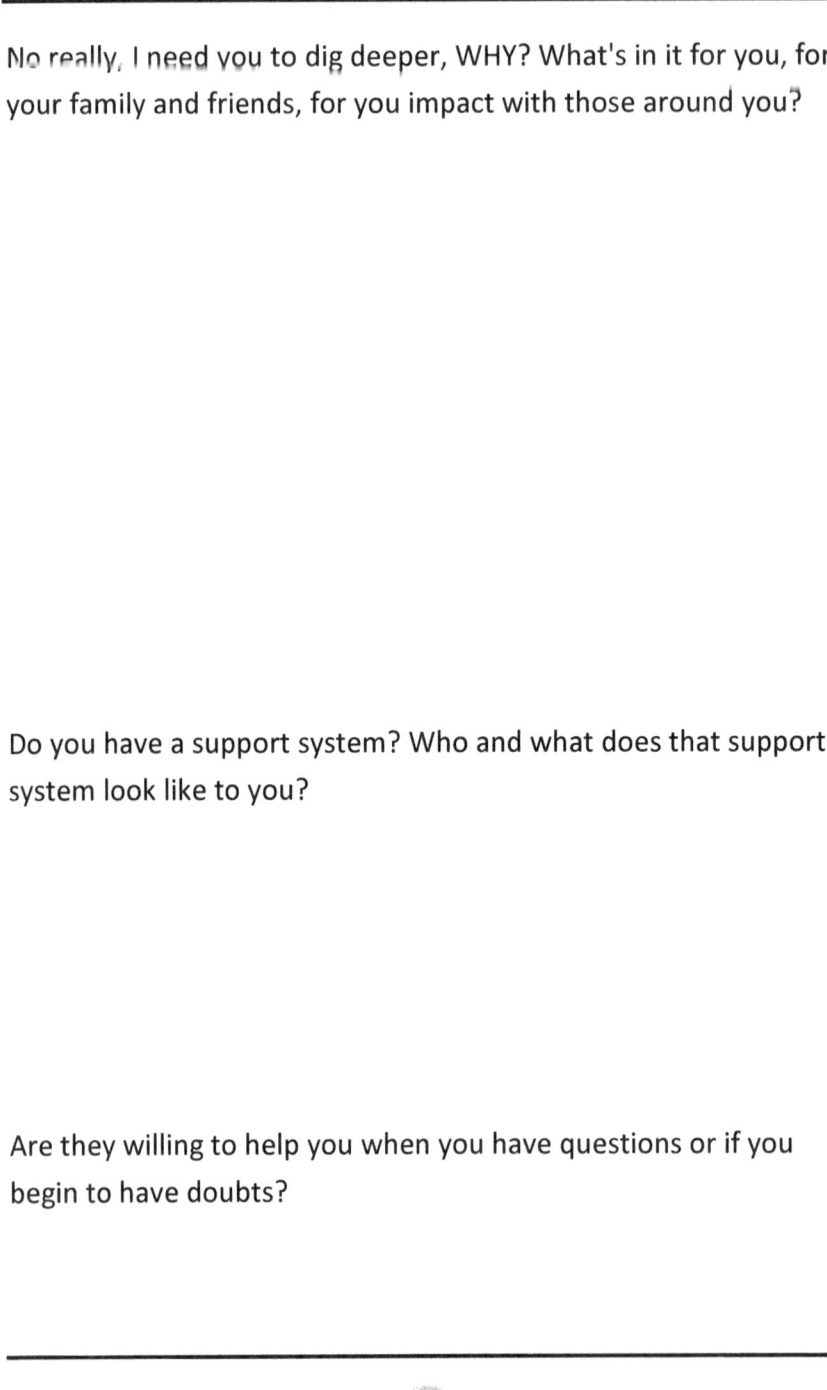

What roadblocks might you face? How will you address those roadblocks?

Where will you purchase your juice or produce? What will you do if specific ingredients are not available?

What about your supplements? Do you have enough on hand or do you need to purchase them?

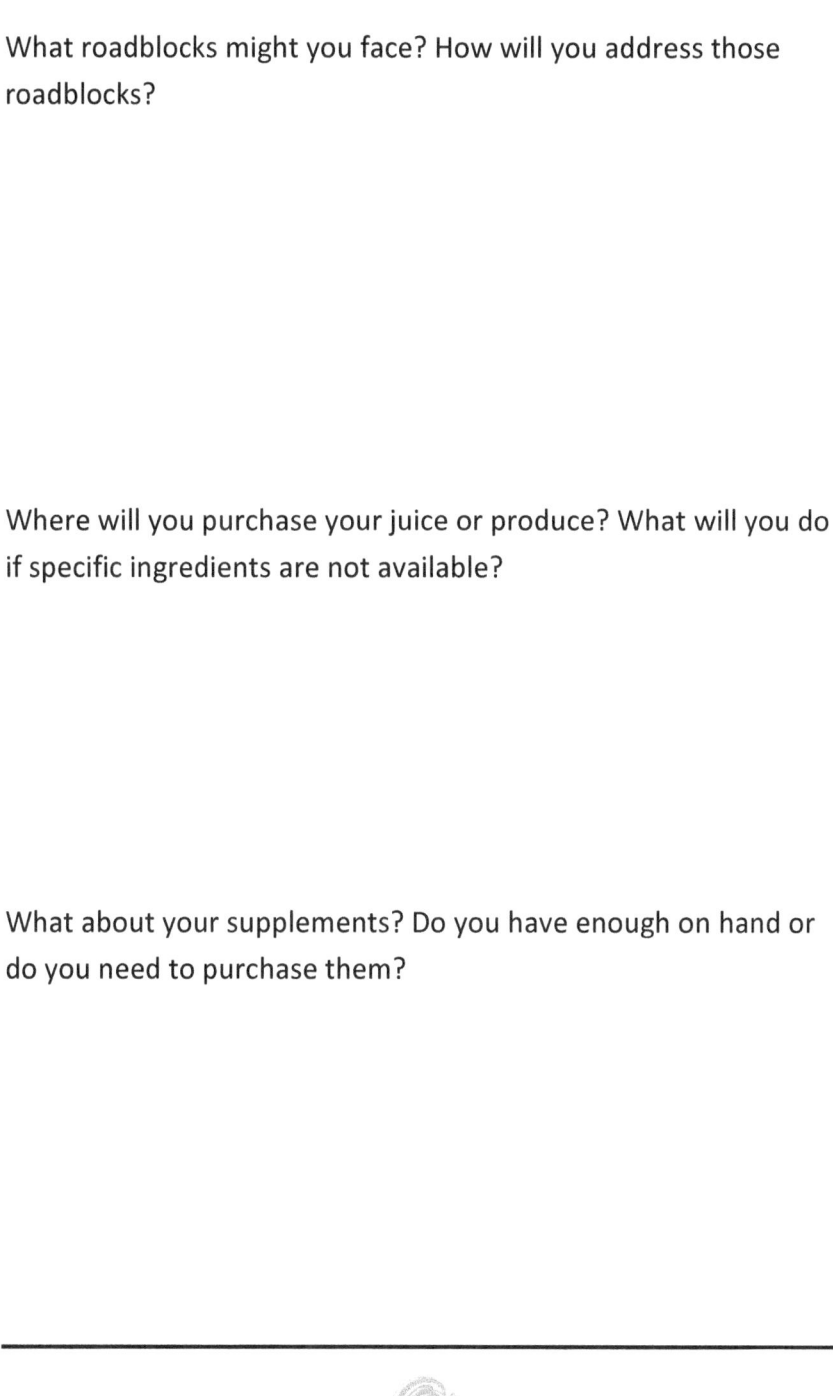

What detox essentials will be part of your fast? (oil pulling, dry skin brushing, etc.) Try to select at least two. Do you have it in stock?

Will you go walking, do yoga, other activities? How often, what time? Do you need to be held accountable?

What spiritual practice will you follow? (meditation, going for a walk, working on a calming hobby)

What self-care will you participate in during your fast? (massage, mani/pedi, etc.)

How will you reward yourself during and after the fast? Will you reward yourself daily or at the completion of the fast? A reward can be a simple as having your favorite juice for dinner, reading a book on a hectic day, or a staycation.

Pre-Juice Fast Day 1

Review previous journal entry.

Do you have produce or juice ready for tomorrow?

Take your measurements. (optional, keep it simple, and don't overwhelm yourself)

How are you feeling emotionally and mentally? This is very important to your success. Try to refrain from writing non-descriptive works such as ok, sad, or happy. Try, I am inspired, overwhelmed, courageous, or worried. Then describe why you feel this way.

Take note of how you feel physically. From head to toe. Your skin, your hair, everything.

What are three things you are grateful for? If you are having a hard time thinking of something, try starting with the simple things of life such as; air, being mobile, sunshine)

Does anything else come to mind that you want to capture?

Review Day 1

Day 1

> "Let food be thy medicine and medicine be thy food." ~
> Hippocrates

Here we are on day one. For some, day one is the most difficult for others day three is the most difficult. Pay attention to your feelings and how you feel physically. Take today one hour at a time, stay in the moment. Breathe often and smile more. Today is a great day, and I believe in you.

During the morning -

Journal for 5 minutes.

Breathe deeply for 1 minute. One of my favorite breathing techniques is to inhale for 6 seconds, hold for 4 seconds, exhale for 6 seconds, hold for 4 seconds, repeat.

Meditate for 5 minutes.

Check-in- How are you feeling emotionally, mentally, spiritually, and physically? Are there any potential roadblocks for today?

What is your affirmation for today? (Example: I quench my thirst for life, I love and approve of myself, I move through life with ease)

What juices will you consume today? How many ounces and how often?

What supplements will you take?

Weigh in. Take your body measurements (optional).

During the day -

Track your mind, body, and soul activities.

How are you feeling?

During the night –

Your first day is done!!! What??? I am super excited for you.
Please be extremely excited for yourself. Okay, now if you didn't
succeed that is okay too. Let's assess, did you drink enough, did
you have enough juice on hand, was it a mental thing. It's okay!
Even if you only traded one meal that is a start. There were
multiple times I started over. Just continue to journal and
reaccess.

What worked well, what did not?

How are you feeling? Physically, emotionally, mentally?

Any "aha" moments?

Write 3 things you are grateful for.

Meditate for 5 minutes.

Day 2

"The food you eat can be either the safest and most powerful form of medicine or the slowest form of poison." ~ Ann Wigmore

Ok, if you completed one day, you can definitely complete two. You know what to do today, you know what to expect, so just breathe and let's get it done!

During the Morning-

Journal for 5 minutes.

Breathe deeply for 1 minute. One of my favorite breathing techniques is to inhale for 6 seconds, hold for 4 seconds, exhale for 6 seconds, hold for 4 seconds, repeat.

Meditate for 5 minutes.

Check-in- How are you feeling emotionally, mentally, spiritually, and physically? Are there any potential roadblocks for today?

What is your affirmation for today? (Example; I quench my thirst for life, I love and approve of myself, I move through life with ease)

What juices will you consume today? How many ounces and how often?

What supplements will you take?

Weigh in. Take your body measurements (optional).

During the day -

Track your mind, body, and soul activities.

How are you feeling?

During the night —

Day 2 done Son! What??? Nice. This is a big accomplishment. You may be flying high or thinking, no really what did I get myself into? Either way, you only have one day to go, and it's an exciting time. You can do it.

What worked well, what did not?

How are you feeling? Physically, emotionally, mentally?

Any "aha" moments?

Write 3 things you are grateful for.

Meditate for 5 minutes.

Day 3

"The best six doctors anywhere and no one can deny it are sunshine, water, rest, air, exercise and diet." ~ Wayne Fields

Exhale… just one more day to go! Monitor your energy level today.

During the morning -

Journal for 5 minutes.

Breathe deeply for 1 minute. One of my favorite breathing techniques is to inhale for 6 seconds, hold for 4 seconds, exhale for 6 seconds, hold for 4 seconds, repeat.

Meditate for 5 minutes.

Check-in- How are you feeling emotionally, mentally, spiritually, and physically? Are there any potential roadblocks for today?

What is your affirmation for today? (Example; I quench my thirst for life, I love and approve of myself, I move through life with ease)

What juices will you consume today? How many ounces and how often?

What supplements will you take?

Weigh in. Take your body measurements (optional).

During the day -

Track your mind, body, and soul activities.

How are you feeling?

During the night –

What worked well, what did not?

How are you feeling? Physically, emotionally, mentally?

Any "aha" moments?

Write 3 things you are grateful for.

Meditate for 5 minutes.

Post Fast

"The greatest wealth is health." ~ Virgil

During the morning

Journal for 5 minutes.

Breathe deeply for 1 minute.

Meditate for 5 minutes.

Check-in- How are you feeling emotionally, mentally, spiritually, and physically?

Weigh in (optional).

Any last thoughts?

Write 3 things you are grateful for.

Notes

Notes

Notes

Notes

Testimonials

Recipes were easy and delicious. The amount of juice kept me from that 3rd-day energy drop. All the materials were easy to follow and very informative. – Curtis T.

Sharon is GREAT! I absolutely love how she dispelled my fears about the juicing fast. I had ZERO worries about how I would handle it because of her! – Tameka A.

Sharon took all of the guesswork out of this program. She made it very easy for me, a beginner, and yet, it was still relevant for juicing veterans. Sharon was easily accessible and helped me throughout the process. Also, I loved the variety of delicious recipes. – Ann E.

After multiple fasting, this particular one put me in a very loving state as well as an empty space to add more beauty and grace. – Leila F.

Resources

http://juiceguru.com

Atlanta-

Living Foods Institute

Arden's Garden

Juice Bar

Kale Me Crazy

Ju-Tox Juice Bar & Wellness Center

Veda Juice

dtox Organic Juice

Rawesome Juicery

Roots Pressed Juice

Bibliography

InnoVision Health Media, Inc. *Alternative Medicine; The Definitive Guide.*

Patrick-Goudreau, Coleen. *Color Me Vegan.*

Ursell, Amanda. *Complete Guide to Healing Foods: Nutritional Healing for Mind and Body.*

Integrated Marketing Services. *Fresh Produce Guide: 300+ fruits, vegetables, and herbs.*

Steven Prussack and Bo Rinaldi. *The Complete Idiot's Guide to Juice Fasting.*

Kordich, Jay. *The Juiceman's Power of Juicing.*

Essene Gospel of Peace Book 1, of the Dead Sea scrolls.

Hay, Louise L. *You Can Heal Your Life.*

Axe, Josh. "Spirulina Benefits: 10 Proven Reasons to Use This Superfood". *Dr. Axe Food is Medicine.* https://draxe.com/spirulina-benefits/

This book was inspired by my experience at the Institute for Integrative Nutrition® (IIN) where I received my training in holistic wellness and health coaching.

IIN offers a truly comprehensive Health Coach Training Program that invites students to deeply explore the things that are most nourishing to them. From the physical aspects of nutrition and eating wholesome foods that work best for each individual person, to the concept of Primary Food – the idea that everything in life including our spirituality, career, relationships, and fitness contribute to our inner and outer health - IIN helped me reach optimal health and balance. This inner journey unleashed the passion that compelled me to share what I've learned and inspire others.

Beyond personal health, IIN offers training in health coaching, as well as business and marketing training. Students who choose to pursue this field professionally, complete the program equipped with the communication skills and branding knowledge they need to create a fulfilling career encouraging and supporting others reach their own health goals.

From renowned wellness experts as Visiting Teachers to the convenience of their online learning platform, this school has changed my life, and I believe it will do the same for you. I invite you to learn more about the Institute for Integrative Nutrition and explore how the Health Coach Training Program can help you transform your life. Feel free to contact me to hear more about my personal experience at www.rawandawesome.com/integrativenutrition, or call (844) 315-8546 to learn more.

ABOUT THE AUTHOR

Sharon Johnson is a Certified Health Coach and Raw Foods Educator. She became a health coach to fulfill her passion of working with busy individuals striving to reach their health goals and happiness through raw living foods, juicing, and lifestyle.

Sharon received her training at Integrative Nutrition in New York City. She received her Living on Live Food Chef Certifications through Alissa Cohen's Raw Teacher Program. She obtained her Juice Guru Certification through Juice Guru.

Sharon leads workshops and retreats on nutrition and offers health and nutrition coaching to individuals and groups.

www.ingramcontent.com/pod-product-compliance
Lightning Source LLC
Chambersburg PA
CBHW070119290526
45789CB00005B/2063